Real Reflections

Real Reflections

Melissa Mathis

authorHOUSE®

AuthorHouse™
1663 Liberty Drive
Bloomington, IN 47403
www.authorhouse.com
Phone: 1-800-839-8640

First published by AuthorHouse   11/07/2011

ISBN: 978-1-4670-9448-1 (sc)
ISBN: 978-1-4670-9449-8 (ebk)

Library of Congress Control Number: 2011919243

Printed in the United States of America

Introduction:

I know, I know, more work! But . . . you want to succeed, don't you? Look around, talk to doctors and dieticians. All of them will say the same thing; keeping a food journal will help you lose weight and keep it off. Of course, we can't just settle for the basic food journal. This is not "just a diet" but an experience; a "taking control and loving our life" experience. We are not just working on the physical, but on *every* aspect of life to create the life you want. There are countless benefits to keeping the journal, if you do it HONESTLY, but one of the best ones is it is a great way to show how far you have come. When I look back on mine, it is amazing to see how hard just a few exercises were for me in the beginning, and to see how many I can do now. Talk about feeling accomplished! We are not looking to conquer the world. We are looking to conquer our fears, insecurities, genetics, depression . . . We can either be our own worst enemy, or our biggest cheerleader. YOU choose!

HOW TO USE MY JOURNAL:

FOOD INTAKE:

Be sure to include what it is, the amount and the calories. I track calories instead of fat because there are many "fat-free" foods that make up for the lack of fat in calories. It is also good to include the time you eat to catch a pattern of when you are eating the most and the reasons behind it.

EXERCISES:

This includes exercises at the gym, workout DVD and exercises at home that you can record the calories burned and the amount of time for the exercises or number, such as fifty sit-ups or twenty minutes on the treadmill. Record calories burned and the amount of calories burned. Also include any active "activities" such as playing with the kids for X amount of minutes or cleaning, also for X amount of minutes. Online is a fountain of information for calories burned for different daily activities.

ACCOMPLISHMENTS:

This is not the exercises you have done. You are already recording that. This could be something from work that you have completed, saying 'no' to the doughnut, passing an exam . . . This is to remind you to FOLLOW through. The gung-ho period is great, but this is especially important when that gung-ho period is over.

"I AM . . .":

It is great to fill out this part in the morning. It could be a full sentence or just one word. Think POSITIVE. I am determined. I am beautiful. I am a success. I am making my dreams come true. I am in control of my life. I am making positive choices . . . and on and on. Re-read this throughout the day. When there is stress, pick up your journal, look at this, read it, feel it, believe it, now . . . live it.

SOMETHING I HAVE DONE FOR MYSELF:

As I wrote in the book, you HAVE to take care of yourself. Again, it is IMPERATIVE that you recharge your batteries. Yes, yes, I agree. You are doing this experience and that is for yourself, and I must say, it is the best thing you can do for yourself, but in this section of your journal you are to do something different that is *just for you!* This could be that you set aside fifteen minutes to have a cup of tea and enjoy a magazine that has been collecting dust. It could be a pedicure. It could be saying no to a task you really don't have time for!

MEASUREMENTS:

This is SO important! Watching one of the weight-loss shows on television as I was going insane working out six days a week, eating healthy, and losing *next to nothing* on the scale, I learned something brilliant. There was a woman who was working her behind off every day and lost only three pounds in two weeks (which, with the workout she was doing, you would have thought she would have lost WAY more), BUT when she was measured, she had lost six inches all over! That is WAY amazing! This part of the journal is important because you are going for the look, not just the number.

Arms: 'R' means right and 'L' means, wow you're smart, yep, left. Most people don't have asymmetrical bodies. One is always bigger than the other. Measure both arms in the same place every time.

Thighs: Refer to above for the 'R' and 'L'. Again, make sure to measure in the same place each time. Freckles are great for place markers!

Under the breast: Women, the easiest way to know this area is the number part of your bra. Don't go with the number on your bra. Measure it yourself!

Across the chest: This is the area with the most coverage in your bra cup. Just think the highest peak, and measure there!

Hips: This is not your saddle bags! This is the area that is above your "area" and, for women, usually the widest area. Just think of where low risers should rest. It is IMPERATIVE that you measure the SAME area each time!

<u>Waist:</u> This is across the belly, at the (hopefully) smallest, curved in part of the stomach. Okay, for me, especially when I first started my experience, there was nothing 'small' or 'curved in' in this section. The belly button is a good marker!

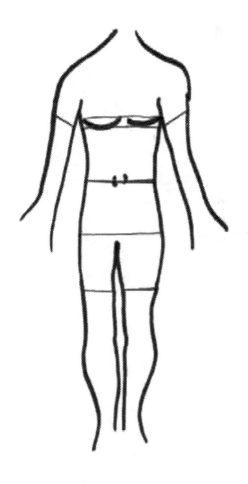

What Sucked/What I Have
Kept Myself From:

_____

_____

_____

_____

_____

_____

_____

_____

_____

_____

_____

_____

_____

_____

_____

_____

_____

_____

_____

_____

_____

_____

_____

_____

_____

_____

_____

_____

_____

Reasons to Stay Fat:

_____
_____
_____
_____
_____
_____
_____
_____
_____
_____
_____
_____
_____
_____
_____
_____
_____
_____
_____
_____
_____
_____
_____
_____
_____
_____
_____

Things I Can Do Instead of AIMLESSLY Eating:

I AM/I HAVE/MY LIFE IS:

(As if you have already achieved all your success,
write it!)

_____
_____
_____
_____
_____
_____
_____
_____
_____
_____
_____
_____
_____
_____
_____
_____
_____
_____
_____
_____
_____
_____
_____
_____
_____

MY ULTIMATE GOAL:

_____

_____

_____

_____

_____

_____

_____

MY GOALS ALONG THE WAY:

(Notice how there are more lines here.
Hmmmmmm . . . I wonder why)

_____

_____

_____

_____

_____

_____

_____

_____

_____

_____

_____

_____

_____

_____

_____

_____

_____

_____

AFTER THE BINGE:

(Emotionally, Physically and Mentally.
Highlight KEY words)

_____

_____

_____

_____

_____

_____

_____

_____

_____

_____

_____

_____

_____

_____

_____

_____

_____

_____

_____

_____

_____

_____

_____

_____

_____

_____

"NORMAL" EATING DAY 1:

WEIGHT: _____
FOOD INTAKE:

_____
_____
_____
_____
_____
_____
_____
_____
_____
_____
_____
_____
_____

ACCOMPLISHMENTS:

_____
_____
_____
_____
_____
_____

EAT HOW YOU NORMALLY EAT!
This is for you to see how much you are REALLY eating. You will refer back to this throughout your experience. Be sure to be honest and measure!

EXERCISES:

_____
_____
_____
_____
_____
_____
_____
_____
_____

I AM _____!

SOMETHING I HAVE DONE FOR MYSELF:

_____
_____
_____
_____
_____

"NORMAL" EATING DAY 2:

WEIGHT: _____

FOOD INTAKE:
_____
_____
_____
_____
_____
_____
_____
_____
_____
_____
_____
_____
_____

ACCOMPLISHMENTS:
_____
_____
_____
_____
_____
_____

EXERCISE HOW YOU ALWAYS DO (OR DON'T)!
Use a pedometer to find out exactly how much you are moving. Don't do more than you normally do. You will be SHOCKED!

EXERCISES:
_____
_____
_____
_____
_____
_____
_____

I AM _____!

SOMETHING I HAVE DONE FOR MYSELF:
_____
_____
_____
_____
_____

DAY 1: CONGRATULATIONS ON YOUR
FIRST DAY OF THE REST OF YOUR LIFE!

WEIGHT: _____   MEASURMENTS:
FOOD INTAKE: UPPER ARMS:
_____   R:_____ L:_____
_____   THIGHS:
_____   R:_____ L:_____
_____   UNDER THE BREAST:
_____   _____
_____   ACROSS THE CHEST:
_____   _____
_____   HIPS:_____
_____   WAIST:_____
_____
_____   EXERCISES:
_____   _____
_____   _____
_____   _____
ACCOMPLISHMENTS: _____
_____   _____
_____   _____
_____   _____
_____   _____
_____   I AM _____!

SOMETHING I HAVE DONE FOR MYSELF:
_____
_____
_____
_____
_____

DAY 2:

WEIGHT: _____

FOOD INTAKE:

_____

_____

_____

_____

_____

_____

_____

_____

_____

_____

_____

_____

Honesty the best policy!
"You lie the loudest when you lie to yourself."
—Author Unknown
If you don't record accurately, *honestly,* you are only hindering your own success!

EXERCISES:

_____

_____

_____

ACCOMPLISHMENTS:

_____

_____

_____

_____

_____

_____

_____

_____

_____

I AM _____ !

SOMETHING I HAVE DONE FOR MYSELF:

_____

_____

_____

_____

_____

DAY 3:

WEIGHT: _____
FOOD INTAKE:
_____
_____
_____
_____
_____
_____
_____
_____
_____
_____
_____
_____

ACCOMPLISHMENTS:
_____
_____
_____
_____
_____
_____

"It is our attitude at the beginning of a difficult task which . . . will affect its successful outcome."— *William James*—If you are going into this experience with a negative attitude, you have already failed. Fix it!

EXERCISES:
_____
_____
_____
_____
_____
_____
_____
_____
_____

I AM _____!

SOMETHING I HAVE DONE FOR MYSELF:
_____
_____
_____
_____
_____

DAY 4:

WEIGHT: _____
FOOD INTAKE:
_____
_____
_____
_____
_____
_____
_____
_____

_____
_____
_____
_____

HELL DAY:
Reality Check!
This is one of the
hardest days. This is
the day that you are
detoxed, regardless of
your diet. This is a 'suck
it up' moment. You have
the strength to do it. It
is in you!

EXERCISES:
_____
_____
_____
_____

ACCOMPLISHMENTS:
_____
_____
_____
_____
_____

_____
_____
_____
_____

I AM _____!

SOMETHING I HAVE DONE FOR MYSELF:
_____
_____
_____
_____
_____

DAY 5:

WEIGHT: _____
FOOD INTAKE:

_____
_____
_____
_____
_____
_____
_____
_____
_____
_____
_____
_____

ACCOMPLISHMENTS:

_____
_____
_____
_____
_____
_____

Let it go!
"The heaviest thing you can carry is a grudge."
—Author Unknown

Remembering the past can motivate you, but keeping your anger for a past hurt only continues to hurt you.

EXERCISES:

_____
_____
_____
_____
_____
_____
_____
_____

I AM _____!

SOMETHING I HAVE DONE FOR MYSELF:

_____
_____
_____
_____
_____

DAY 6:

WEIGHT: _____
FOOD INTAKE:
_____
_____
_____
_____
_____
_____
_____
_____
_____
_____
_____
_____
_____

ACCOMPLISHMENTS:
_____
_____
_____
_____
_____
_____

Talking to yourself?

If you answered no, this is the wrong answer! Tell yourself daily, not how amazing you are going to be, but how amazing you already are! Find the miracles in yourself!

EXERCISES:
_____
_____
_____
_____
_____
_____
_____
_____

I AM _____!

SOMETHING I HAVE DONE FOR MYSELF:
_____
_____
_____
_____
_____

DAY 7:

WEIGHT: _____
FOOD INTAKE:
_____
_____
_____
_____
_____
_____
_____
_____
_____
_____
_____
_____
_____

ACCOMPLISHMENTS:
_____
_____
_____
_____
_____
_____

"It is better to offer no excuse than a bad one."
—George Washington
Stop making excuses for yourself! Accept your blame, and your responsibility, and then you will be able to accept your kudos for your success!

EXERCISES:
_____
_____
_____
_____
_____
_____
_____

I AM _____!

SOMETHING I HAVE DONE FOR MYSELF:
_____
_____
_____
_____
_____

DAY 8:

WEIGHT: _____
FOOD INTAKE:
_____
_____
_____
_____
_____
_____
_____
_____
_____
_____
_____
_____

Looking back at me!
Hello? Are you looking,
ACTUALLY looking at
your reflection when
you pass your mirrors?
Owning exercise
equipment doesn't make
you lose weight, USING
it does. Same with your
mirrors!

EXERCISES:
_____
_____
_____
_____

ACCOMPLISHMENTS:
_____
_____
_____
_____
_____
_____

I AM _____!

SOMETHING I HAVE DONE FOR MYSELF:
_____
_____
_____
_____
_____

DAY 9:

WEIGHT: _____
FOOD INTAKE:

_____
_____
_____
_____
_____
_____
_____
_____
_____
_____
_____

ACCOMPLISHMENTS:

_____
_____
_____
_____
_____
_____

"Plan for gradual improvement, not spectacular leaps . . . A slow and steady stream of water will erode the hardest rock."
—David Campbell Ph.D
Step by step, my friend, step by step!

EXERCISES:

_____
_____
_____
_____
_____
_____
_____
_____

I AM _____!

SOMETHING I HAVE DONE FOR MYSELF:

_____
_____
_____
_____
_____

DAY 10:

<u>WEIGHT:</u> _____
<u>FOOD INTAKE:</u>
_____
_____
_____
_____
_____
_____
_____
_____
_____
_____
_____
_____
_____

<u>ACCOMPLISHMENTS:</u>
_____
_____
_____
_____
_____
_____

Your get-up-and-go got up and left!
Your gung-ho-ness is gone. *Amazingly* you aren't at your goal yet! You're doing *everything* you are supposed to do and, you're STILL NOT THERE?!? Well, did you gain it all in ten days . . . ?

<u>EXERCISES:</u>
_____
_____
_____
_____
_____
_____
_____

I AM _____!

SOMETHING I HAVE DONE FOR MYSELF:
_____
_____
_____
_____
_____

DAY 11:

WEIGHT: _____

FOOD INTAKE:
_____
_____
_____
_____
_____
_____
_____
_____
_____
_____
_____
_____

ACCOMPLISHMENTS:
_____
_____
_____
_____
_____

"You have to learn the rules of the game. And then you have to play better than anyone else."—Einstein

This book contains the rules of this game. Learn well! KICK BUTT! You can, and will, win!

EXERCISES:
_____
_____
_____
_____
_____
_____
_____
_____

I AM _____!

SOMETHING I HAVE DONE FOR MYSELF:
_____
_____
_____
_____
_____

DAY 12:

WEIGHT: _____
FOOD INTAKE:
_____
_____
_____
_____
_____
_____
_____
_____
_____
_____
_____
_____

ACCOMPLISHMENTS:
_____
_____
_____
_____
_____

"If you get a second chance, grab it with both hands. If it changes your life, let it. Nobody said life would be easy, they just promised it would be worth it"
—Author Unknown
Don't lose your chance at the life you want!

EXERCISES:
_____
_____
_____
_____
_____
_____
_____
_____

I AM _____!

SOMETHING I HAVE DONE FOR MYSELF:
_____
_____
_____
_____
_____

DAY 13:

WEIGHT: _____
FOOD INTAKE:
_____
_____
_____
_____
_____
_____
_____
_____
_____
_____
_____
_____
_____

ACCOMPLISHMENTS:
_____
_____
_____
_____
_____
_____

"Before you embark on a journey of revenge, dig two graves."
—Confucius
You have to let go of anger. This is probably harder than anything else in this experience. If you hold onto anger, you will never move forward.

EXERCISES:
_____
_____
_____
_____
_____
_____
_____
_____

I AM _____!

SOMETHING I HAVE DONE FOR MYSELF:
_____
_____
_____
_____
_____

DAY 14: CONGRATULATIONS! YOU HAVE OFFICIALLY

MADE IT THROUGH THE HARDEST WEEKS!

WEIGHT: _____

FOOD INTAKE:

_____

_____

_____

_____

_____

_____

_____

_____

_____

_____

_____

_____

ACCOMPLISHMENTS:

_____

_____

_____

_____

_____

MEASURMENTS:

UPPER ARMS:

R:_____ L:_____

THIGHS:

R:_____ L:_____

UNDER THE BREAST:

_____

ACROSS THE CHEST:

_____

HIPS:_____

WAIST:_____

EXERCISES:

_____

_____

_____

_____

_____

_____

_____

I AM _____!

SOMETHING I HAVE DONE FOR MYSELF:

_____

_____

_____

_____

_____

DAY 15:

WEIGHT: _____
FOOD INTAKE:
_____
_____
_____
_____
_____
_____
_____
_____
_____
_____
_____
_____
_____
_____

ACCOMPLISHMENTS:
_____
_____
_____
_____
_____
_____

You are starting to see results! Yea!
Your pants are a bit easier to button. Be sure to write the 'little' things you notice. It's all the little successes along the way. You may now proceed to the happy bootie dance!

EXERCISES:

_____
_____
_____
_____
_____
_____
_____

I AM _____!

SOMETHING I HAVE DONE FOR MYSELF:
_____
_____
_____
_____
_____

DAY 16:

WEIGHT: _____
FOOD INTAKE:
_____
_____
_____
_____
_____
_____
_____
_____
_____
_____
_____
_____

ACCOMPLISHMENTS:
_____
_____
_____
_____
_____
_____

"Our achievements
of today are but the
sum of our thoughts
of yesterday. You
are today where the
thoughts of yesterday
have brought you and
will be tomorrow, where
the thoughts of today
take you."—Pascal

EXERCISES:
_____
_____
_____
_____
_____
_____
_____
_____

I AM _____!

SOMETHING I HAVE DONE FOR MYSELF:
_____
_____
_____
_____
_____

DAY 17:

WEIGHT: _____
FOOD INTAKE:
_____
_____
_____
_____
_____
_____
_____
_____
_____
_____
_____
_____
_____
_____

ACCOMPLISHMENTS:
_____
_____
_____
_____
_____

Have an attitude of gratitude! Make a list of 50 things you are thankful for, even something as small as a coffee break. Hey, you woke up today, didn't you? Be sure to refer back to this list often! Look in the back of your journal for this page!

EXERCISES:

_____
_____
_____
_____
_____
_____
_____
_____

I AM _____!

SOMETHING I HAVE DONE FOR MYSELF:
_____
_____
_____
_____
_____

DAY 18:

WEIGHT: _____
FOOD INTAKE:
_____
_____
_____
_____
_____
_____
_____
_____
_____
_____
_____
_____

ACCOMPLISHMENTS:
_____
_____
_____
_____
_____
_____

"If you could kick the person in the pants responsible for most of your trouble, you wouldn't sit for a month"
—Theodore Roosevelt
You have to accept your responsibility for your lot in life!

EXERCISES:
_____
_____
_____
_____
_____
_____
_____
_____
_____

I AM _____!

SOMETHING I HAVE DONE FOR MYSELF:
_____
_____
_____
_____
_____

DAY 19:

WEIGHT: _____

FOOD INTAKE:

_____

_____

_____

_____

_____

_____

_____

_____

_____

_____

_____

_____

_____

Not-so-random act of kindness:
Of course, this experience is ALL ABOUT YOU, but, helping others actually gives you a high. What is something you have done to help another?

ACCOMPLISHMENTS:

_____

_____

_____

_____

_____

_____

EXERCISES:

_____

_____

_____

_____

_____

_____

_____

_____

I AM _____!

SOMETHING I HAVE DONE FOR MYSELF:

_____

_____

_____

_____

_____

DAY 20:

WEIGHT: _____
FOOD INTAKE:
_____
_____
_____
_____
_____
_____
_____
_____
_____
_____
_____
_____

ACCOMPLISHMENTS:
_____
_____
_____
_____
_____
_____

Your attitude is going to
determine your success.
Anything you go into
with a negative attitude
is not going to succeed.
Check the bad attitude
at the door and enter
with the idea that you
are already a success!

EXERCISES:
_____
_____
_____
_____
_____
_____
_____
_____
_____

I AM _____!

SOMETHING I HAVE DONE FOR MYSELF:
_____
_____
_____
_____
_____

DAY 21:

WEIGHT: _____
FOOD INTAKE:

_____
_____
_____
_____
_____
_____
_____
_____
_____
_____
_____
_____
_____

ACCOMPLISHMENTS:

_____
_____
_____
_____
_____
_____

Creating Healthy Habits:

I have heard after 21 days of doing something, it becomes a habit. What are some tips that are now habits?

EXERCISES:

_____
_____
_____
_____
_____
_____
_____
_____
_____

I AM _____!

SOMETHING I HAVE DONE FOR MYSELF:

_____
_____
_____
_____
_____

DAY 22:

__WEIGHT:__ _____
__FOOD INTAKE:__
_____
_____
_____
_____
_____
_____
_____
_____
_____
_____
_____
_____

__ACCOMPLISHMENTS:__
_____
_____
_____
_____
_____

You can either play the blame game, saying, "I couldn't because . . ." or you can choose to take control of your life and direct it towards the direction you want to go. As always, the choice is yours.

__EXERCISES:__
_____
_____
_____
_____
_____
_____
_____
_____
I AM _____!

__SOMETHING I HAVE DONE FOR MYSELF:__
_____
_____
_____
_____
_____

DAY 23:

WEIGHT: _____
FOOD INTAKE:
_____
_____
_____
_____
_____
_____
_____
_____
_____
_____
_____
_____

ACCOMPLISHMENTS:
_____
_____
_____
_____
_____
_____

Augh! Not AGAIN!
Are you sick of the
same diet? Sick of the
same fruits and veggies?
Are the results not what
you thought it would
be? Now is the time
to change it up and try
something new!

EXERCISES:
_____
_____
_____
_____
_____
_____
_____
_____
_____

I AM _____!

SOMETHING I HAVE DONE FOR MYSELF:
_____
_____
_____
_____
_____

DAY 24:

WEIGHT: _____
FOOD INTAKE:
_____
_____
_____
_____
_____
_____
_____
_____
_____
_____
_____
_____

"It is not the mountain we conquer but ourselves."
—Edmund Hillary
Weight loss is not just about what we eat and exercise, it is about conquering the problems that got us fat in the first place.

EXERCISES:

_____
_____
_____
_____

ACCOMPLISHMENTS:
_____
_____
_____
_____
_____
_____

_____
_____
_____
_____

I AM _____!

SOMETHING I HAVE DONE FOR MYSELF:
_____
_____
_____
_____
_____

DAY 25:

WEIGHT: _____

FOOD INTAKE:
_____
_____
_____
_____
_____
_____
_____
_____
_____
_____
_____
_____

ACCOMPLISHMENTS:
_____
_____
_____
_____
_____

Give what you want to get!
When was the last
time you REALLY
complimented someone;
a sincere compliment?
There is no such thing
as a self-less act. This
WILL benefit you. Go.
Now. Compliment!

EXERCISES:
_____
_____
_____
_____
_____
_____
_____
_____
_____

I AM _____!

SOMETHING I HAVE DONE FOR MYSELF:
_____
_____
_____
_____
_____

DAY 26:

WEIGHT: _____
FOOD INTAKE:
_____
_____
_____
_____
_____
_____
_____
_____
_____
_____
_____
_____

ACCOMPLISHMENTS:
_____
_____
_____
_____
_____
_____

"Nothing will work unless you do."—Maya Angelou You have to work to reach your goal. If you think you are going to just wake up thin with no effort, WAKE UP! You have to work to achieve success. Get to it!

EXERCISES:
_____
_____
_____
_____
_____
_____
_____
_____

I AM _____!

SOMETHING I HAVE DONE FOR MYSELF:
_____
_____
_____
_____
_____

DAY 27:

WEIGHT: _____
FOOD INTAKE:
_____
_____
_____
_____
_____
_____
_____
_____
_____
_____
_____
_____
_____

ACCOMPLISHMENTS:
_____
_____
_____
_____
_____
_____

"We all find ourselves in situations that seem hopeless. We have the choice to do nothing or take action."
—Catherine Pulsifer
Being fat feels hopeless, out of control, but you are in control of your life. You choose!

EXERCISES:
_____
_____
_____
_____
_____
_____
_____
_____
_____

I AM _____!

SOMETHING I HAVE DONE FOR MYSELF:
_____
_____
_____
_____
_____

DAY 28: WOW! NEARLY A MONTH ALREADY! HOW YA FEELIN'?

WEIGHT: _____

FOOD INTAKE:
_____
_____
_____
_____
_____
_____
_____
_____
_____
_____

ACCOMPLISHMENTS:
_____
_____
_____
_____
_____

MEASURMENTS:
UPPER ARMS:
R:_____ L:_____
THIGHS:
R:_____ L:_____
UNDER THE BREAST:
_____
ACROSS THE CHEST:
_____
HIPS:_____
WAIST:_____

EXERCISES:
_____
_____
_____
_____
_____
_____
_____
_____

I AM _____!

SOMETHING I HAVE DONE FOR MYSELF:
_____
_____
_____
_____
_____

DAY 29:

WEIGHT: _____
FOOD INTAKE:
_____
_____
_____
_____
_____
_____
_____
_____
_____
_____
_____
_____
_____

ACCOMPLISHMENTS:
_____
_____
_____
_____
_____
_____

REVIEW WHAT SUCKED!
Remember that list
you made of how it
sucked to be fat? Read
it. Again. And again.
Know you are taking
charge and control, and
most amazingly, truly
beginning to
LIVE your life!

EXERCISES:
_____
_____
_____
_____
_____
_____
_____
_____
_____
_____

I AM _____!

SOMETHING I HAVE DONE FOR MYSELF:
_____
_____
_____
_____
_____

DAY 30:

WEIGHT: _____

FOOD INTAKE:

_____

_____

_____

_____

_____

_____

_____

_____

_____

_____

_____

ACCOMPLISHMENTS:

_____

_____

_____

_____

_____

BE WISE!

Knowledge: Knowing the right thing to do.

Wisdom: Doing what you know you should do.

You make the choice!

EXERCISES:

_____

_____

_____

_____

_____

_____

_____

_____

I AM _____!

SOMETHING I HAVE DONE FOR MYSELF:

_____

_____

_____

_____

_____

43

DAY 31:

WEIGHT: _____
FOOD INTAKE:
_____
_____
_____
_____
_____
_____
_____
_____
_____
_____
_____
_____
_____
_____

ACCOMPLISHMENTS:
_____
_____
_____
_____
_____
_____

"I had to pick myself up and get on with it, do it all over again, only even better this time."
—Sam Walton
Even if you have an "out of control" day, a bad day, do better the next time!

EXERCISES:
_____
_____
_____
_____
_____
_____
_____
_____

I AM _____!

SOMETHING I HAVE DONE FOR MYSELF:
_____
_____
_____
_____
_____

DAY 32:

WEIGHT: _____
FOOD INTAKE:
_____
_____
_____
_____
_____
_____
_____
_____
_____
_____
_____
_____

ACCOMPLISHMENTS:
_____
_____
_____
_____
_____
_____

"If you'll not settle for anything less than your best, you will be amazed at what you can accomplish in your life,"
—Vince Lombardi
Never give anything less than your best for your life!

EXERCISES:
_____
_____
_____
_____
_____
_____
_____
_____

I AM _____!

SOMETHING I HAVE DONE FOR MYSELF:
_____
_____
_____
_____
_____

DAY 33:

WEIGHT: _____
FOOD INTAKE:
_____
_____
_____
_____
_____
_____
_____
_____
_____
_____
_____
_____
_____

ACCOMPLISHMENTS:
_____
_____
_____
_____
_____
_____

"There is no failure except in no longer trying."
—Elbert Hubbard
This might not be easy to attempt, but being fat isn't easy either. Push yourself as you have never pushed before!

EXERCISES:
_____
_____
_____
_____
_____
_____
_____
_____
_____

I AM _____!

SOMETHING I HAVE DONE FOR MYSELF:
_____
_____
_____
_____
_____

DAY 34:

WEIGHT: _____
FOOD INTAKE:
_____
_____
_____
_____
_____
_____
_____
_____
_____
_____
_____

"Many people die at twenty-five and aren't buried until they are seventy-five."
—Benjamin Franklin
Live each moment of your life, your experience, even before you have reached your ultimate goal!

ACCOMPLISHMENTS:
_____
_____
_____
_____
_____
_____

EXERCISES:
_____
_____
_____
_____
_____
_____
_____
_____

I AM _____!

SOMETHING I HAVE DONE FOR MYSELF:
_____
_____
_____
_____
_____

47

DAY 35:

__WEIGHT:__ _____
__FOOD INTAKE:__
_____
_____
_____
_____
_____
_____
_____
_____
_____
_____
_____
_____
_____

__ACCOMPLISHMENTS:__
_____
_____
_____
_____
_____

"When you dance, your purpose is not to get to a certain place on the floor. It's to enjoy each step along the way."
—Waye Dyer
Make and *enjoy* your smaller goals along the way!

__EXERCISES:__
_____
_____
_____
_____
_____
_____
_____
_____

__I AM__ _____!

__SOMETHING I HAVE DONE FOR MYSELF:__
_____
_____
_____
_____
_____

DAY 36:

WEIGHT: _____
FOOD INTAKE:
_____
_____
_____
_____
_____
_____
_____
_____
_____
_____
_____
_____
_____

ACCOMPLISHMENTS:
_____
_____
_____
_____
_____
_____

Augh!!!
You mean you have pushed through an entire month and you're *still* not at your goal yet? But wait, look at how much better you are today than day 1. See the progress?
More to come!!!

EXERCISES:
_____
_____
_____
_____
_____
_____
_____

I AM _____!

SOMETHING I HAVE DONE FOR MYSELF:
_____
_____
_____
_____
_____

DAY 37:

WEIGHT: _____
FOOD INTAKE:
_____
_____
_____
_____
_____
_____
_____
_____
_____
_____
_____
_____
_____

ACCOMPLISHMENTS:
_____
_____
_____
_____
_____
_____

"Every horse thinks its
own pack heaviest."
—Thomas Fuller
Everybody has their
burdens. Don't think
your life is so much
harder than people
who have succeeded.
They have just pushed
through, and so will you!

EXERCISES:
_____
_____
_____
_____
_____
_____
_____

I AM _____!

SOMETHING I HAVE DONE FOR MYSELF:
_____
_____
_____
_____
_____

DAY 38:

WEIGHT: _____
FOOD INTAKE:
_____
_____
_____
_____
_____
_____
_____
_____
_____
_____
_____
_____

"A healthy mind is a healthy body."
Juvenal (55ad-127 AD)
I put in the date of his life to show you that even then they knew the "secret". No diet is going to work if you don't heal your mind!

EXERCISES:
_____
_____
_____
_____

ACCOMPLISHMENTS:
_____
_____
_____
_____
_____
_____
_____

I AM _____!

SOMETHING I HAVE DONE FOR MYSELF:
_____
_____
_____
_____
_____

DAY 39:

WEIGHT: _____
FOOD INTAKE:
_____
_____
_____
_____
_____
_____
_____
_____
_____
_____
_____
_____
_____
_____

ACCOMPLISHMENTS:
_____
_____
_____
_____
_____
_____

Kiddie time!
Remember to carry
kid's utensils with you
when out eating with
friends. They may look
at you strangely now,
but imagine how they
will look at you when you
have reached your goal!

EXERCISES:
_____
_____
_____
_____
_____
_____
_____
_____
_____
_____

I AM _____!

SOMETHING I HAVE DONE FOR MYSELF:
_____
_____
_____
_____
_____

DAY 40:

WEIGHT: _____
FOOD INTAKE:

_____
_____
_____
_____
_____
_____
_____
_____
_____
_____
_____
_____

ACCOMPLISHMENTS:

_____
_____
_____
_____
_____
_____

PUT THE CHIPS
DOWN!
I know, I know. It has
been so long since you
were able to just eat
without thinking about
it. Yeah, and, look at
where that mindless
eating got you to . . . Put.
It. Down! GREAT JOB!

EXERCISES:

_____
_____
_____
_____
_____
_____
_____
_____

I AM _____!

SOMETHING I HAVE DONE FOR MYSELF:

_____
_____
_____
_____
_____

DAY 41:

WEIGHT: _____
FOOD INTAKE:
_____
_____
_____
_____
_____
_____
_____
_____
_____
_____
_____
_____

ACCOMPLISHMENTS:
_____
_____
_____
_____
_____
_____

"We can throw stones, complain about them, stumble on them, climb over them, or build with them."—W.A. Ward
You can complain about your problems or find a way to use them to your benefit. Find a way to use them!

EXERCISES:
_____
_____
_____
_____
_____
_____
_____
_____
I AM _____!

SOMETHING I HAVE DONE FOR MYSELF:
_____
_____
_____
_____
_____

DAY 42: LOVIN' IT AND HATIN' IT . . .
BUT, IT IS WORKING! KEEP PUSHING!

WEIGHT: _____

FOOD INTAKE:

_____

_____

_____

_____

_____

_____

_____

_____

_____

_____

_____

_____

ACCOMPLISHMENTS:

_____

_____

_____

_____

_____

MEASURMENTS:

UPPER ARMS:

R:_____ L:_____

THIGHS:

R:_____ L:_____

UNDER THE BREAST:

_____

ACROSS THE CHEST:

_____

HIPS:_____

WAIST:_____

EXERCISES:

_____

_____

_____

_____

_____

_____

_____

_____

I AM _____!

SOMETHING I HAVE DONE FOR MYSELF:

_____

_____

_____

_____

_____

DAY 43:

<u>WEIGHT:</u> _____

<u>FOOD INTAKE:</u>

_____

_____

_____

_____

_____

_____

_____

_____

_____

_____

"Be kind, for everyone you meet is fighting a hard battle."—Plato Remember, you are not the only one whose life is not perfect. Another may have it even harder. Be kind and hope for that kindness in return!

<u>EXERCISES:</u>

_____

_____

_____

_____

<u>ACCOMPLISHMENTS:</u>

_____

_____

_____

_____

_____

_____

I AM _____!

SOMETHING I HAVE DONE FOR MYSELF:

_____

_____

_____

_____

_____

DAY 44:

WEIGHT: _____
FOOD INTAKE:
_____
_____
_____
_____
_____
_____
_____
_____
_____
_____
_____

"Improvement begins
with 'I'"
—Arnold H. Glasgow
Changing your life begins
with YOU! If you don't
change your perception
of health and weight
loss and dealing with
stress, you lose. Start
with "I".

EXERCISES:

ACCOMPLISHMENTS:
_____
_____
_____
_____
_____
_____

_____
_____
_____
_____
_____
_____

I AM _____!

SOMETHING I HAVE DONE FOR MYSELF:
_____
_____
_____
_____
_____

DAY 45:

<u>WEIGHT:</u> _____
<u>FOOD INTAKE:</u>

_____
_____
_____
_____
_____
_____
_____
_____
_____
_____
_____

<u>ACCOMPLISHMENTS:</u>

_____
_____
_____
_____
_____
_____

"I never knew a man
come to greatness or
eminence who lay abed
late in the morning."
—Jonathan Swift
So . . . remember when
I told you to get up ten
minutes earlier? Well,
have you been doing it?

<u>EXERCISES:</u>

_____
_____
_____
_____
_____
_____
_____
_____

I AM _____!

SOMETHING I HAVE DONE FOR MYSELF:

_____
_____
_____
_____
_____

DAY 46:

WEIGHT: _____
FOOD INTAKE:
_____
_____
_____
_____
_____
_____
_____
_____
_____
_____
_____

ACCOMPLISHMENTS:
_____
_____
_____
_____
_____

"If I had permitted my failures, or what seemed to me at the time a lack of success, to discourage me, I cannot see any way in which I would have ever made progress."—Coolidge Allow for your own success!

EXERCISES:
_____
_____
_____
_____
_____
_____
_____

I AM _____!

SOMETHING I HAVE DONE FOR MYSELF:
_____
_____
_____
_____
_____

DAY 47:

WEIGHT: _____

FOOD INTAKE:

_____
_____
_____
_____
_____
_____
_____
_____
_____
_____
_____
_____
_____

ACCOMPLISHMENTS:

_____
_____
_____
_____
_____
_____

"There is but one cause of human failure. And that is man's lack of faith in his true Self."—William James You have to trust in your ability to achieve anything you set your mind to. Trust in your own strength!

EXERCISES:

_____
_____
_____
_____
_____
_____
_____
_____

I AM _____!

SOMETHING I HAVE DONE FOR MYSELF:

_____
_____
_____
_____
_____

DAY 48:

WEIGHT: _____
FOOD INTAKE:

_____
_____
_____
_____
_____
_____
_____
_____
_____
_____
_____
_____

ACCOMPLISHMENTS:

_____
_____
_____
_____
_____
_____

"If you don't like
something, change it.
If you can't change it,
change your attitude.
Don't complain."

—Maya Angelou

Need I say more?

EXERCISES:

_____
_____
_____
_____
_____
_____
_____
_____

I AM _____!

SOMETHING I HAVE DONE FOR MYSELF:

_____
_____
_____
_____
_____

DAY 49:

WEIGHT: _____
FOOD INTAKE:
_____
_____
_____
_____
_____
_____
_____
_____
_____
_____
_____
_____
_____

ACCOMPLISHMENTS:
_____
_____
_____
_____
_____

"It's not whether you get knocked down, it's whether you get back up."
—Vince Lombardi
You're human. You are going to have slip-ups. Are you going to let that keep you down?
Hello? NO!

EXERCISES:
_____
_____
_____
_____
_____
_____
_____
_____

I AM _____!

SOMETHING I HAVE DONE FOR MYSELF:
_____
_____
_____
_____
_____

DAY 50:

WEIGHT: _____
FOOD INTAKE:
_____
_____
_____
_____
_____
_____
_____
_____
_____
_____
_____
_____

ACCOMPLISHMENTS:
_____
_____
_____
_____
_____
_____

Where's the elevator?
Feels like you are
climbing a HUGE flight
of stairs! There is no
elevator, Dearheart.
Turn around and enjoy
the view from where
you are right now.
You have a bit to go,
but have come so far!
CONGRATULATIONS!
EXERCISES:
_____
_____
_____
_____
_____
_____
_____
_____

I AM _____!

SOMETHING I HAVE DONE FOR MYSELF:
_____
_____
_____
_____
_____

DAY 51:

WEIGHT: _____
FOOD INTAKE:

_____
_____
_____
_____
_____
_____
_____
_____
_____
_____
_____
_____

ACCOMPLISHMENTS:

_____
_____
_____
_____
_____

"If you're walking down the right path and you're willing to keep walking, eventually you'll make progress."
—President Obama
If you are tired of trying, take one more step, then one more.

EXERCISES:

_____
_____
_____
_____
_____
_____
_____
_____

I AM _____!

SOMETHING I HAVE DONE FOR MYSELF:

_____
_____
_____
_____
_____

DAY 52:

WEIGHT: _____
FOOD INTAKE:
_____
_____
_____
_____
_____
_____
_____
_____
_____
_____
_____
_____
_____

ACCOMPLISHMENTS:
_____
_____
_____
_____
_____
_____

"Don't worry about the world coming to an end today. It's already tomorrow in Australia." Charles Schulz As stated in the book, learn to deal with stress. Stress makes you fat. Period. Deal with it!

EXERCISES:
_____
_____
_____
_____
_____
_____
_____
_____

I AM _____!

SOMETHING I HAVE DONE FOR MYSELF:
_____
_____
_____
_____
_____

DAY 53:

WEIGHT: _____
FOOD INTAKE:
_____
_____
_____
_____
_____
_____
_____
_____
_____
_____
_____
_____
_____

ACCOMPLISHMENTS:
_____
_____
_____
_____
_____
_____

"Even if you are on the right track, you'll get run over if you just sit there."
—Will Rogers
Don't stop. Never give in. One foot after the other. Left, then right. Then left again. Repeat.

EXERCISES:
_____
_____
_____
_____
_____
_____
_____
_____
_____

I AM _____!

SOMETHING I HAVE DONE FOR MYSELF:
_____
_____
_____
_____
_____

DAY 54:

WEIGHT: _____
FOOD INTAKE:

_____
_____
_____
_____
_____
_____
_____

_____
_____
_____
_____
_____

ACCOMPLISHMENTS:

_____
_____
_____
_____
_____

So, I never told you this experience was going to be easy. I said it would be WORTH it. Dig deep in yourself and find your strength. You are stronger than you know. Now show yourself just how strong you are!

EXERCISES:

_____
_____
_____
_____
_____
_____
_____
_____

I AM _____!

SOMETHING I HAVE DONE FOR MYSELF:

_____
_____
_____
_____
_____

DAY 55:

WEIGHT: _____
FOOD INTAKE:
_____
_____
_____
_____
_____
_____
_____
_____
_____
_____
_____
_____
_____

ACCOMPLISHMENTS:
_____
_____
_____
_____
_____
_____

After the BINGE!
Re-read what you wrote
after the binge. It's
been a long time since
you have felt like that,
huh? NEVER forget
where you came from.
The moment you forget,
the moment you **LOSE**.
Always appreciate!

EXERCISES:
_____
_____
_____
_____
_____
_____
_____
_____

I AM _____!

SOMETHING I HAVE DONE FOR MYSELF:
_____
_____
_____
_____
_____

DAY 56: YOU HAVE ACTUALLY STUCK TO THIS FOR THIS LONG? YOU ROCK!

WEIGHT: _____

FOOD INTAKE:
_____
_____
_____
_____
_____
_____
_____
_____
_____
_____
_____

ACCOMPLISHMENTS:
_____
_____
_____
_____
_____

MEASURMENTS:

UPPER ARMS:
R:_____ L:_____
THIGHS:
R:_____ L:_____
UNDER THE BREAST:
_____

ACROSS THE CHEST:
_____

HIPS:_____
WAIST:_____

EXERCISES:
_____
_____
_____
_____
_____
_____
_____

I AM _____!

SOMETHING I HAVE DONE FOR MYSELF:
_____
_____
_____
_____
_____

DAY 57:

WEIGHT: _____
FOOD INTAKE:
_____
_____
_____
_____
_____
_____
_____
_____
_____

Take a long, hard look at yourself!
Take a good look in the mirror. Note any difference-not just measurements but, WOW, you have cheekbones, that you can see! A jaw line? Visible? Enjoy all the changes! You Rock!

EXERCISES:
_____
_____
_____
_____

ACCOMPLISHMENTS:
_____
_____
_____
_____
_____
_____

_____
_____
_____
_____

I AM _____!

SOMETHING I HAVE DONE FOR MYSELF:
_____
_____
_____
_____
_____

DAY 58:

__WEIGHT:__ _____

__FOOD INTAKE:__

_____

_____

_____

_____

_____

_____

_____

_____

_____

_____

_____

_____

__ACCOMPLISHMENTS:__

_____

_____

_____

_____

_____

"The successful man will profit from his mistakes and try again in a different way."
—Dale Carnegie
Wow! You mean to tell me that even successful people make mistakes? Oh, yeah, we're human. Keep trying!

__EXERCISES:__

_____

_____

_____

_____

_____

_____

_____

__I AM__ _____!

SOMETHING I HAVE DONE FOR MYSELF:

_____

_____

_____

_____

_____

DAY 59:

WEIGHT: _____
FOOD INTAKE:
_____
_____
_____
_____
_____
_____
_____
_____
_____
_____
_____
_____
_____

ACCOMPLISHMENTS:
_____
_____
_____
_____
_____
_____

Excuse to shop!
Buy, or cut out of a
magazine an outfit you
want to wear when
you are at your goal. I
tacked it to my bedroom
wall. Visualize how
awesome you will feel
when you are able
to fit it!

EXERCISES:
_____
_____
_____
_____
_____
_____
_____
_____

I AM _____!

SOMETHING I HAVE DONE FOR MYSELF:
_____
_____
_____
_____
_____

DAY 60:

WEIGHT: _____
FOOD INTAKE:

_____

_____

_____

_____

_____

_____

_____

_____

_____

_____

_____

_____

ACCOMPLISHMENTS:

_____

_____

_____

_____

_____

Say Cheese!
Smiling, the free tummy
tuck! Smile like you
mean it! Remember, even
if it is a fake smile, it
will fool your brain into
thinking you really are
happy! More happy =
Less munching!

EXERCISES:

_____

_____

_____

_____

_____

_____

_____

I AM _____!

SOMETHING I HAVE DONE FOR MYSELF:

_____

_____

_____

_____

_____

DAY 61:

WEIGHT: _____
FOOD INTAKE:
_____
_____
_____
_____
_____
_____
_____
_____
_____
_____
_____
_____

ACCOMPLISHMENTS:
_____
_____
_____
_____
_____

Hey! I can stretch my arms! How are your clothes feeling? Sleeves looser? Do you have to keep pulling up your pants? Congratulations! Notice ALL the 'small' changes. Be sure to appreciate it and want it more!

EXERCISES:
_____
_____
_____
_____
_____
_____
_____

I AM _____!

SOMETHING I HAVE DONE FOR MYSELF:
_____
_____
_____
_____
_____

DAY 62:

WEIGHT: _____
FOOD INTAKE:
_____
_____
_____
_____
_____
_____
_____
_____
_____
_____
_____
_____

You have to make the
choice within yourself
to succeed. If you don't
like your situation, then
change it. Change begins
within yourself. When
you change inside, the
outside will follow!

EXERCISES:
_____
_____
_____
_____

ACCOMPLISHMENTS:
_____
_____
_____
_____
_____

_____
_____
_____
_____

I AM _____!

SOMETHING I HAVE DONE FOR MYSELF:
_____
_____
_____
_____
_____

Melissa Mathis

DAY 63:

WEIGHT: _____
FOOD INTAKE:
_____
_____
_____
_____
_____
_____
_____
_____
_____
_____
_____

ACCOMPLISHMENTS:
_____
_____
_____
_____
_____
_____

Fake it 'til you make it!
Are you practicing who
you want to become?
Are you paying attention
to people who are
already where you want
to be? Create yourself.
You are in control of
your life!

EXERCISES:
_____
_____
_____
_____
_____
_____
_____
_____

I AM _____!

SOMETHING I HAVE DONE FOR MYSELF:
_____
_____
_____
_____
_____

DAY 64:

WEIGHT: _____
FOOD INTAKE:
_____
_____
_____
_____
_____
_____
_____
_____
_____
_____
_____
_____

Thin chicks & the green-eyed monster! "Do they *appreciate* being thin?" Who cares? All that matters is, do *you* appreciate where you are now? Look at them and realize one day, someone will be looking at you!

EXERCISES:
_____
_____
_____

ACCOMPLISHMENTS:
_____
_____
_____
_____
_____

_____
_____
_____
_____

I AM _____!

SOMETHING I HAVE DONE FOR MYSELF:
_____
_____
_____
_____
_____

DAY 65:

WEIGHT: _____
FOOD INTAKE:
_____
_____
_____
_____
_____
_____
_____
_____
_____
_____
_____
_____
_____

ACCOMPLISHMENTS:
_____
_____
_____
_____
_____
_____

Have you tried?
Have you tried that new workout class you have always wanted to, but have been too afraid or ashamed to try? Now is the time to try something new! Be sure to learn to laugh at yourself!

EXERCISES:
_____
_____
_____
_____
_____
_____
_____

I AM _____!

SOMETHING I HAVE DONE FOR MYSELF:
_____
_____
_____
_____
_____

DAY 66:

WEIGHT: _____

FOOD INTAKE:

_____
_____
_____
_____
_____
_____
_____
_____
_____
_____
_____
_____

How's work?
Are you seeing the
difference in the rest
of your life? Do you
see you are getting
more accomplished than
before? Getting more
done at work and still
have energy? Keep going!

ACCOMPLISHMENTS:

_____
_____
_____
_____
_____

EXERCISES:

_____
_____
_____
_____
_____
_____
_____
_____

I AM _____!

SOMETHING I HAVE DONE FOR MYSELF:

_____
_____
_____
_____
_____

DAY 67:

WEIGHT: _____
FOOD INTAKE:

_____
_____
_____
_____
_____
_____
_____
_____

_____
_____
_____
_____
_____

ACCOMPLISHMENTS:

_____
_____
_____
_____
_____

"I could not . . . be content to take my place by the fireside and look on. Life was meant to be lived. One must never, for whatever reason, turn his back on life."
—Eleanor Roosevelt
Permission to enjoy your life!

EXERCISES:

_____
_____
_____
_____
_____
_____
_____
_____
_____

I AM _____!

SOMETHING I HAVE DONE FOR MYSELF:

_____
_____
_____
_____
_____

DAY 68:

WEIGHT: _____
FOOD INTAKE:
_____
_____
_____
_____
_____
_____
_____
_____
_____
_____
_____
_____

ACCOMPLISHMENTS:
_____
_____
_____
_____
_____
_____

No pain, ALL weight gain!
Are your workouts
getting easier? Great!
Now, you have to step it
up. If it gets too easy,
if you don't feel *some*
soreness, you aren't
going to lose more.
PUSH IT!

EXERCISES:
_____
_____
_____
_____
_____
_____
_____
_____

I AM _____!

SOMETHING I HAVE DONE FOR MYSELF:
_____
_____
_____
_____
_____

DAY 69:

WEIGHT: _____
FOOD INTAKE:
_____
_____
_____
_____
_____
_____
_____
_____
_____
_____
_____
_____

ACCOMPLISHMENTS:
_____
_____
_____
_____
_____

"Our bodies communicate to us clearly and specifically, if we are willing to listen to them."
—Shakti Gawain

Uh . . . Hello? PAY ATTENTION!

EXERCISES:
_____
_____
_____
_____
_____
_____
_____

I AM _____!

SOMETHING I HAVE DONE FOR MYSELF:
_____
_____
_____
_____
_____

DAY 70: RESULTS ARE REALLY BEGINNING TO SHOW! DON'T QUIT NOW!

WEIGHT: _____

FOOD INTAKE:

_____

_____

_____

_____

_____

_____

_____

_____

_____

_____

_____

_____

ACCOMPLISHMENTS:

_____

_____

_____

_____

_____

MEASURMENTS:

UPPER ARMS:

R:_____ L:_____

THIGHS:

R:_____ L:_____

UNDER THE BREAST:

_____

ACROSS THE CHEST:

_____

HIPS:_____

WAIST:_____

EXERCISES:

_____

_____

_____

_____

_____

_____

_____

_____

I AM _____!

SOMETHING I HAVE DONE FOR MYSELF:

_____

_____

_____

_____

_____

DAY 71:

WEIGHT: _____
FOOD INTAKE:

_____
_____
_____
_____
_____
_____
_____
_____
_____
_____
_____
_____
_____

Not so much!
Finding that your 'usual' cravings aren't so usual anymore? Not hungry as often? Don't forget to eat, especially breakfast, or your metabolism will slow down!

EXERCISES:

_____
_____
_____
_____
_____
_____
_____
_____

ACCOMPLISHMENTS:

_____
_____
_____
_____
_____
_____

I AM _____!

SOMETHING I HAVE DONE FOR MYSELF:

_____
_____
_____
_____
_____

DAY 72:

WEIGHT: _____
FOOD INTAKE:

_____

_____

_____

_____

_____

_____

_____

_____

_____

_____

_____

_____

ACCOMPLISHMENTS:

_____

_____

_____

_____

_____

"We should not look back unless it is to derive useful lessons from past errors, and for the purpose of profiting by dearly bought experience."
—George Washington
Look back on how far you have come!

EXERCISES:

_____

_____

_____

_____

_____

_____

_____

I AM _____!

SOMETHING I HAVE DONE FOR MYSELF:

_____

_____

_____

_____

_____

DAY 73:

WEIGHT: _____
FOOD INTAKE:
_____
_____
_____
_____
_____
_____
_____
_____
_____
_____
_____
_____
_____

ACCOMPLISHMENTS:
_____
_____
_____
_____
_____
_____

Surprise!
Isn't it amazing how you have more confidence now? Have you even realized it? Notice you are doing things you would never have tried before? Awesome, isn't it?

EXERCISES:
_____
_____
_____
_____
_____
_____
_____

I AM _____!

SOMETHING I HAVE DONE FOR MYSELF:
_____
_____
_____
_____
_____

DAY 74:

WEIGHT: _____
FOOD INTAKE:
_____
_____
_____
_____
_____
_____
_____
_____
_____
_____
_____
_____

ACCOMPLISHMENTS:
_____
_____
_____
_____
_____
_____

"Study the past if you would define the future."—Confucius Review your journal entries for the days you were eating how you 'normally' ate before this experience. See how different you're eating now?

EXERCISES:
_____
_____
_____
_____
_____
_____
_____
_____
_____

I AM _____!

SOMETHING I HAVE DONE FOR MYSELF:
_____
_____
_____
_____
_____

DAY 75:

WEIGHT: _____
FOOD INTAKE:
_____
_____
_____
_____
_____
_____
_____
_____
_____
_____
_____
_____
_____

ACCOMPLISHMENTS:
_____
_____
_____
_____
_____
_____

Hellooo Girdie!
You may now need to buy a new girdle or undershirt. This is GREAT! This means you are losing inches! Just remember! The whole point of these are to be tight to aid your awareness!

EXERCISES:

_____
_____
_____
_____
_____
_____
_____
_____
_____

I AM _____!

SOMETHING I HAVE DONE FOR MYSELF:
_____
_____
_____
_____
_____

DAY 76:

WEIGHT: _____
FOOD INTAKE:
_____
_____
_____
_____
_____
_____
_____
_____
_____
_____
_____
_____
_____

ACCOMPLISHMENTS:
_____
_____
_____
_____
_____
_____
_____

What have you done for me lately?
What have you rewarded yourself with recently? Are you really appreciating all your successes? Notice this theme of appreciation? Hmmm . . . Maybe it's IMPORTANT!

EXERCISES:
_____
_____
_____
_____
_____
_____
_____
_____
_____

I AM _____!

SOMETHING I HAVE DONE FOR MYSELF:
_____
_____
_____
_____
_____

DAY 77:

WEIGHT: _____

FOOD INTAKE:

_____

_____

_____

_____

_____

_____

_____

_____

_____

_____

_____

_____

_____

Quit Camping!
So . . . have you gotten
rid of the tents yet?
Still taking yourself
out in draw-strings?
You're getting there, I
know, but make sure you
aren't covering all your
success!

EXERCISES:

_____

_____

_____

_____

ACCOMPLISHMENTS:

_____

_____

_____

_____

_____

_____

_____

_____

_____

I AM _____!

SOMETHING I HAVE DONE FOR MYSELF:

_____

_____

_____

_____

_____

DAY 78:

<u>WEIGHT:</u> _____
<u>FOOD INTAKE:</u>

_____
_____
_____
_____
_____
_____
_____
_____
_____
_____
_____
_____

<u>ACCOMPLISHMENTS:</u>

_____
_____
_____
_____
_____

Now which one?
By now you may have
tried several different
diets. Which one worked
the best for you? Which
one has been the easiest
one to follow? Mix it up
and find what works
for you!

<u>EXERCISES:</u>

_____
_____
_____
_____
_____
_____
_____
_____

I AM _____!

SOMETHING I HAVE DONE FOR MYSELF:

_____
_____
_____
_____
_____

DAY 79:

WEIGHT: _____
FOOD INTAKE:
_____
_____
_____
_____
_____
_____
_____
_____
_____
_____
_____
_____
_____

ACCOMPLISHMENTS:
_____
_____
_____
_____
_____
_____

"I finally realized that being grateful to my body was key to giving more love to myself."
—Oprah Winfrey
Wow! See how successful she is? Hmmmm . . . Maybe she's onto something!

EXERCISES:
_____
_____
_____
_____
_____
_____
_____
_____

I AM _____!

SOMETHING I HAVE DONE FOR MYSELF:
_____
_____
_____
_____
_____

DAY 80:

WEIGHT: _____

FOOD INTAKE:

_____
_____
_____
_____
_____
_____
_____
_____
_____
_____
_____
_____
_____

ACCOMPLISHMENTS:

_____
_____
_____
_____
_____

"Each body has its art . . ."
—Gwendolyn Brooks
Look into your
mirror; *really* look
into the mirror and
see the beauty of you,
the real you.
Write it down
and smile!

EXERCISES:

_____
_____
_____
_____
_____
_____
_____
_____

I AM _____!

SOMETHING I HAVE DONE FOR MYSELF:

_____
_____
_____
_____
_____

DAY 81:

WEIGHT: _____
FOOD INTAKE:

_____

_____

_____

_____

_____

_____

_____

_____

_____

_____

_____

ACCOMPLISHMENTS:

_____

_____

_____

_____

_____

"The minds first step
to self-awareness must
be through the body."
—George Sheehan
Um . . . isn't that kinda
what I've been trying
to tell you? The fat
is trying tell you. Find
what the *real* prob. is.

EXERCISES:

_____

_____

_____

_____

_____

_____

_____

_____

I AM _____!

SOMETHING I HAVE DONE FOR MYSELF:

_____

_____

_____

_____

_____

DAY 82:

<u>WEIGHT:</u> _____
<u>FOOD INTAKE:</u>

_____
_____
_____
_____
_____
_____
_____
_____

_____
_____
_____
_____

<u>ACCOMPLISHMENTS:</u>

_____
_____
_____
_____
_____

"Motivation comes from the goals you truly desire to accomplish and your commitment to do whatever necessary to accomplish the goals."—Russ Mallard Commit yourself to making your life the most amazing life it can be!

<u>EXERCISES:</u>

_____
_____
_____
_____
_____
_____
_____
_____

I AM _____!

SOMETHING I HAVE DONE FOR MYSELF:

_____
_____
_____
_____
_____

DAY 83:

WEIGHT: _____
FOOD INTAKE:

_____
_____
_____
_____
_____
_____
_____
_____
_____
_____
_____
_____

Think again!
Only one more day to
the end of this journal,
but it isn't the end
for you! You are just
beginning! Your LIFE is
just beginning! Read and
re-read the book *and*
your journal. Enjoy!

EXERCISES:

_____
_____
_____
_____
_____

ACCOMPLISHMENTS:

_____
_____
_____
_____
_____

_____
_____
_____
_____

I AM _____!

SOMETHING I HAVE DONE FOR MYSELF:

_____
_____
_____
_____
_____

DAY 84: THIS MAY BE THE LAST DAY OF YOUR

JOURNAL, BUT THE BEGINNING OF YOUR JOURNEY!

DO NOT STOP NOW!

WEIGHT: _____   MEASURMENTS:

FOOD INTAKE: UPPER ARMS:

_____   R:_____ L:_____

_____   THIGHS:

_____   R:_____ L:_____

_____   UNDER THE BREAST:

_____   _____

_____   ACROSS THE CHEST:

_____   _____

_____   HIPS:_____

_____   WAIST:_____

_____

_____   EXERCISES:

_____   _____

ACCOMPLISHMENTS: _____

_____   _____

_____   _____

_____   _____

_____   _____

_____   I AM _____!

SOMETHING I HAVE DONE FOR MYSELF:

_____

_____

_____

_____

_____

50 THINGS I AM THANKFUL FOR: